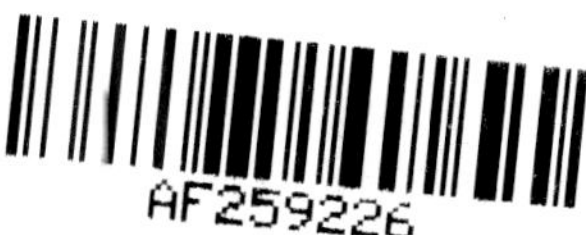

This journal belongs to

____

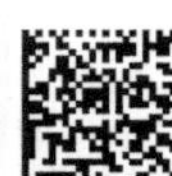

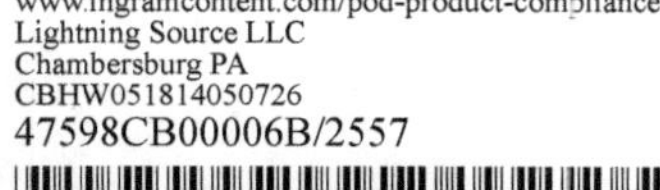
9 781797 432793